ISBN: 9781674434155

101
WEIGHT LOSS
TIPS and
'Secrets'

Compiled by

NoPaperPress staff

CONTENTS

101 Weight Loss

Tips and 'Secrets'

Compiled by the NoPaperPress™ staff

The following are offered to help you loose weight in a healthy and natural way. Use the tips that apply to you and can best help you succeed. Good luck!

Basic Diet Tips & Secrets

1) A reducing diet is best supervised by a physician. This is especially true when a great deal of weight needs to be lost, or if you have an ailment or a history of medical problems.

2) Understand that the only sure way to slim down for keeps is to eat less and exercise more. There are no safe short cuts or miracle methods for taking off weight.

3) Successful weight loss and subsequent weight maintenance requires knowledge, desire and discipline. Avoid the latest fad diets. Instead, take the time to develop a true understanding of weight control and then change your eating and activity habits accordingly.

4) Consistently choose healthy foods, avoid

harmful foods and large portions and exercise regularly. Nothing else will work over the long haul.

5) What constitutes a good reducing diet? A good weight loss diet must provide you with an <u>understanding</u> of weight control as well as the knowledge you need to reduce your weight to the desired level.

6) A good reducing diet must also help you remain healthy while you are losing weight.

7) In addition, a good reducing diet must lead you to a healthier way of eating and exercising that will help you, in the long term, keep off the weight you have lost.

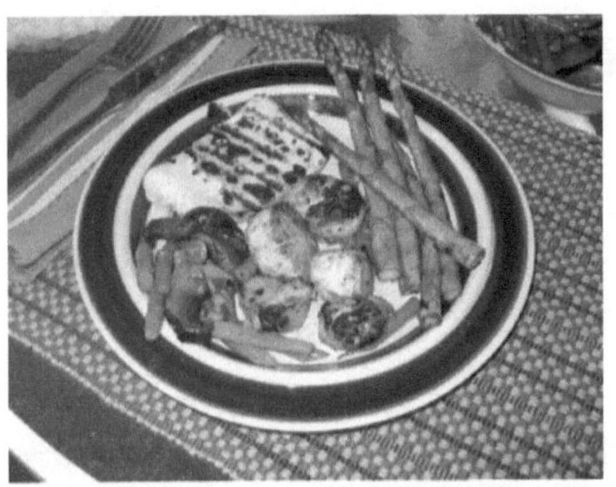

8) First, ask yourself: "Why am I overweight?" What are the main reasons? Do you eat too much of everything? Too much dessert? Drink too much beer? Is your only exercise walking from the TV to the fridge? Determine the why and then focus on those one or two problem areas. Sometimes it's that simple.

9) Experts agree that whether you are trying to lose weight or just maintain your weight, it's calories that count.   It doesn't matter what foods the calories are from – to lose weight you must eat fewer calories than you burn. Calories count!   Not carbs, not Weight Watchers points. Calories – period!

10) Weight control can be thought of as supply and demand. You lose weight if you supply your body with fewer calories than your activities demand. (In this case, your body uses energy you stored as fat to make up the calorie difference.)

11) Weight loss occurs when your food energy intake is less than the total energy you expend. This difference in calories is referred to as your calorie deficit.

12) How much weight you lose depends on the magnitude of your calorie deficit. To lose one pound requires a deficit of approximately 3,500 Calories.

13) Use Body Mass Index, or BMI, to determine what you should weigh. Your BMI is calculated by dividing your weight in kilograms by the square of your height in meters. (See "Weight Control – U.S. Edition," published by NoPaperPress.com for a convenient, easy-to-use chart).

14) Given two people the same age, gender and activity level, and on the same reducing diet, the heavier person will lose weight faster than the thinner person.

15) Given a male and female, the same age, weight, activity level and on the same reducing diet, the man will lose weight faster than the woman. This is due to the fact that women have less muscle and therefore lower basal metabolic rates than men. Hence, a woman must eat less than a man to lose the same amount of weight.

16) Given two individuals, the same gender, weight and activity level, the younger person will lose weight faster than the older person.

17) If your caloric intake is constant over the years you will slowly gain weight as you age. This is because your basal metabolic rate decreases as you

advance in age, and most people tend not to be as active as they get older.

18) If you are overweight start on a weight loss diet now because it will only become more difficult to lose weight as you get older.

19) If your caloric intake on a weight-loss diet is constant, your rate of weight loss will decrease with time. So if you want to lose weight at a constant rate over time, you must eat slightly less (or exercise harder) as you lose weight.

20) Inevitably, everyone on a diet hits a exasperating weight-loss plateau. The only way to bust through the plateau is to reduce your caloric intake and/or to step up your exercise intensity.

21) Slow weight loss is healthier, is more likely to be permanent, and is easier to sustain over the long haul. So when it comes to weight loss, don't be in a hurry!

22) A very important weight-profile parameter is your waist-to-hip ratio. Health risks for heart attack and stroke increase considerably for men with a ratio above 1.0 and for women with a ratio above 0.8. To calculate your ratio, measure your waist size (at its narrowest circumference) and divide it by your hip size (at its widest section).

23) The general weight-loss rule is "last on first off." When you lose weight, it normally it will come off in the reverse order of where you gained it.   And there is

not much you can do about that. There is no food, no exercise, no magic pill that will cause your body to lose fat in one place rather than another.

24) To determine your frame size, circle your wrist with your thumb and third finger. If the tips of your fingers overlap, you have a small frame. If they just touch you are medium, and if they don't touch you have a large frame.

Basic Eating Tips & Secrets

25) The diet of most Americans is not very healthy. Most of us consume too many calories, saturated fat, trans fat, cholesterol, added sugars and salt.

26) An understanding of nutrition is not only vital for good health but also helps you control your weight in the long term.

27) Keep a daily food log to record everything you eat. For some people it really works wonders.

28) Read food labels carefully to know what's in the food you buy and eat, and to avoid foods with hidden calories.

29) "Eat Slowly." This is especially vital when you're trying to lose weight. If you're someone who eats fast, you're not giving yourself a chance to feel full. While everyone else is still eating, you either sit and pick, or you have seconds, taking in extra calories you could avoid if you would just slow down.

30) Drink lots of water – about 8 glasses per day. Try adding a slice of lemon to make it more interesting. Often, when you think you're hungry, you're just thirsty. So, next time you reach for a snack, drink some water first and see if that does it for you.

31) Hunger is your body's way of telling you that you need fuel, that is calories. When you're done eating, you should feel satisfied – but not stuffed.

32) Remember your stomach is about the size of your fist. So it doesn't take much food to fill it comfortably.

Food & Calorie Tips & Secrets

33) All foods are a combination of water, carbohydrate, protein, fat and fiber. Knowing this can lead to a better understanding of why a food has a particular caloric value.

34) When on a diet, an awareness of the caloric value (per ounce) of some basic foods can really be helpful.

35) Fat (lard) has the highest calorie per ounce value – about 260.   Sugar (a pure carbohydrate) at 110 Calories per ounce is near the middle of the calorie spectrum.

36) Water and fiber contain no calories – that is zero Calories per ounce.

37) One dilemma for dieters is judging portion size. It makes no sense to worry about whether a cut of lean meat has 70 or 80 Calories per ounce if you have no idea whether the portion you are eating weighs four or ten ounces. To be successful, learn to estimate portion sizes with reasonable accuracy.

38) Judging the weight of meat or poultry is one of the most important parts of any diet. As a guide, four ounces of meat or poultry is about the size of a slice of bread: 4 x 4 x ¼ inch.

Practical Eating Tips & Secrets

39) To control portion size, that is the amount of food you eat, use a salad plate instead of a dinner plate.

40) Eat the low-cal items on your plate first. Start

with a broth soup, then the salad and veggies. By the time you get to the higher calorie meat and starch you'll be almost full and will eat less of them.

41) Studies show people who eat 5 to 6 mini-meals and snacks a day don't feel as hungry and are better able to control their appetite and their weight.

42) Foods loaded with flavor stimulate your taste buds and are more satisfying. So add herbs and spices to your food for a flavor boost and you might not eat as much.

43) When on a diet simple is better. Why? Because simple, uncomplicated meals usually contain fewer "hidden calories" than more elaborate dishes.

44) Fat-free isn't always your best bet.   Low fat doesn't necessarily mean low calorie! Most often sugar is substituted for fat and the calorie total remains the same or even higher. Instead, look for low-calorie or reduced-calorie foods.

45) Fat-free (skim) milk is the exception. To cut calories, switch to 1-percent milk or even better fat-free milk.

46) Hot or cold cereal topped with fruit, and fat-free milk makes a nutritious, relatively low-calorie meal anytime.

47) For a quick low-cal meal, try a peanut butter sandwich on whole wheat bread with a glass of 1-percent milk and an apple.

48) Keep several bags of your favorite frozen vegetables on hand. Mix any combination, microwave, and top with your favorite light salad dressing. Makes a great low-cal meal.

49) For another quick low-cal meal, try a Lean Cuisine or Healthy Choice frozen entree with a salad and a glass of 1-percent milk.

50) Keep lean sandwich fixings on hand (whole-wheat bread, sliced turkey, reduced-fat cheese, lettuce, tomatoes and mustard).

51) Try to use mustard on a sandwich instead of mayo.

52) For a healthy and relatively low-calorie meal, buy a veggie sandwich on whole-wheat bread at Subway.

53) If you hate veggies, eat plenty of fruit instead. Fruit is just about as healthy and low-calorie as vegetables.

54) To prevent a diet from becoming monotonous, after a few weeks try exchanging or substituting foods – a technique used by dieticians. Exchanging a food listed in a diet for another food with approximately equal caloric value and nutritional content is the foundation of a successful long-term diet.

55) Handle occasional overeating by compensating. To do this, estimate how far you have strayed from your weight-loss diet and then make amends at the next opportunity (usually the next meal or two) – by eating less.

56) Learn to change your eating habits to meet changing activity levels – that is don't eat as much when you're activity level declines.

<u>Binge Eating Avoidance Tips & Secrets</u>

57) Most nutritionists recommend that you eat a substantial breakfast because then you'll likely eat less the remainder of the day.

58) Eating late at night doesn't by itself cause weight gain. Because it's the total number of calories that count – not when you eat them.

59) But don't "snack" yourself fat. You can easily munch 600 calories of chips and dips while watching late-night TV.

60) A majority of people who struggle with night-binge eating are those who skip meals during the day. Make sure you eat breakfast, lunch, and dinner.

61) To avoid night-binge eating, change your evening routine. Rather than watching TV get into a hobby that will occupy your mind and hands.

62) Post a notice on your kitchen and refrigerator doors: "Closed After Dinner."

63) Brush your teeth immediately after dinner to discourage you from continued eating.

<u>**Eating in Restaurants Tips & Secrets**</u>

64) Eating in a restaurant can be a challenge because most restaurant portions are huge, and can easily total

more than 1,500 Calories.   So, when you're in a restaurant decide how much to eat – and take the remainder home. A good rule of thumb is to eat half and bring the rest home.

65) When you're eating out, consider ordering children's portions or a small sandwich as a way to trim calories and get the size of your meals under control.

66) In a restaurant, consider ordering two appetizers (one should be low-calorie) instead of an entrée, and always request sauces and dressings on the side.

67) For even better calorie control, eat at home rather than in a restaurant.

68) To save calories and money, instead of eating out, bring your lunch to work.

Party Tips & Secrets

69) Before you go to a party, have a very small meal or snack to take the edge off your appetite and make it easier to resist high-calorie goodies.

70) At a party, don't stand near temptation – the food and the bar!   You'll probably eat and drink less.

71) If you host a dinner party, when company leaves, have them take some of the leftover food (particularly the dessert) with them – or take the leftovers to work the next day.

<u>**Drinking Tips & Secrets**</u>

72) Beware of alcoholic beverages. Beer has about 13 Calories per ounce, wine has 25 Calories per ounce and whiskey has a whopping 71 Calories per ounce!

73) Drink alcoholic beverages in moderation and try to restrict any alcoholic drinking to weekends.

74) Stop drinking your calories.   Alcoholic drinks, fancy coffees, regular soda, and even fruit juice are high in calories – but they don't make you feel full.

75) Dilute fruit juices, such as apple juice, orange juice, etc. with water. This does cut the flavor slightly but really reduces the calorie content.

<u>**Dessert Tips & Secrets**</u>

76)   Don't have sweets in your home.   This makes them easier to resist.   Out of sight, out of mind!

77) Instead of sweets, for a delicious, healthy, low-calorie dessert have a low-cal smoothie, or sliced fruit over low-fat or fat-free yogurt.

78) On the other hand, not eating your favorite foods sometimes triggers "rebound" overeating. Even on a diet you can still enjoy your favorite foods – but do so in moderation.

79) If you must have sweets, allow about 150 calories per day
for your favorite sweet – which amounts to roughly one ounce of chocolate, half a slice of cake, or ½ cup of ice cream.

<u>**Nutrition Tips & Secrets**</u>

80) According to a study published in the Journal of Food Chemistry, broccoli, spinach, kale, Brussels sprouts and other dark green vegetables have the highest cancer-fighting potential found in produce. And all are super-low calorie foods.

81) Steaming in a microwave is an excellent way to cook veggies so they retain nutrients.   Another advantage is that steaming adds no fat (calories) or sodium.

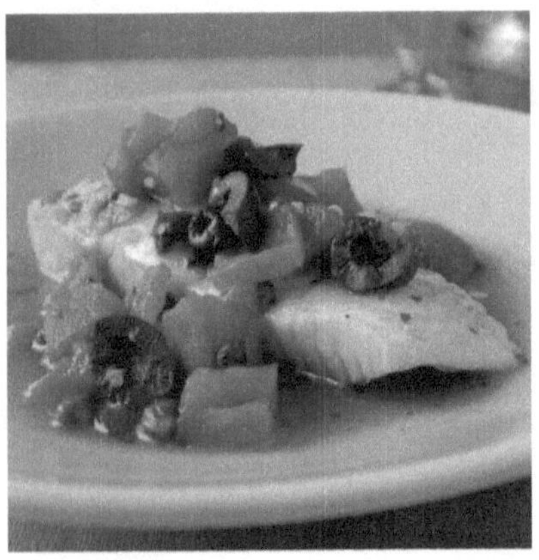

82) Protein foods make you feel full longer and a can help you avoid overeating.

83) Free-range animals get more exercise and eat a natural diet, so their meat is usually lower in fat and calories than farm-raised cattle.

Exercise Tips & Secrets

84) Muscle is active tissue, fat is not. The more muscle you have, the more calories you burn. Muscle uses a significant number of calories every day for repair and rebuilding, giving your metabolism a boost even when you're resting. So make sure strengthening exercises (like weight lifting) are part of your workout.

85) Because strengthening exercises work a muscle until it's fatigued, take a day off between strength workouts so your muscles can recover, repair and rebuild.

86) You can workout anywhere you have extra space, in a bedroom, basement, garage, or attic.   A set of variable (adjustable) weight dumbbells and a small weight bench don't take up much room and are all you need for a home-based gym.

87) Working out at home has some significant advantages. Your workout takes less time because you don't have to drive back and forth to a fitness facility; and you have the
flexibility of dividing your workout into small time segments to fit your day, and working out at home is less expensive.

88) Bear in mind, knowledge and the discipline to workout regularly are far more important than fancy equipment.

89) Avoid injury by warming up and cooling down slowly.

90) Avoid injury by building up exercise intensity gradually over many weeks, months.

91) Stay Busy. Most people will do anything to avoid work, housework, yard work, exercise, etc.   But any kind of work burns a lot more calories than just sitting. Whatever it is you are avoiding – just go and do it!

92)   Buy a pedometer and start walking.   For the average person 2,100 steps amounts to walking about one mile. A Harvard study has shown that 8,000 to 10,000 step per day promotes weight loss.

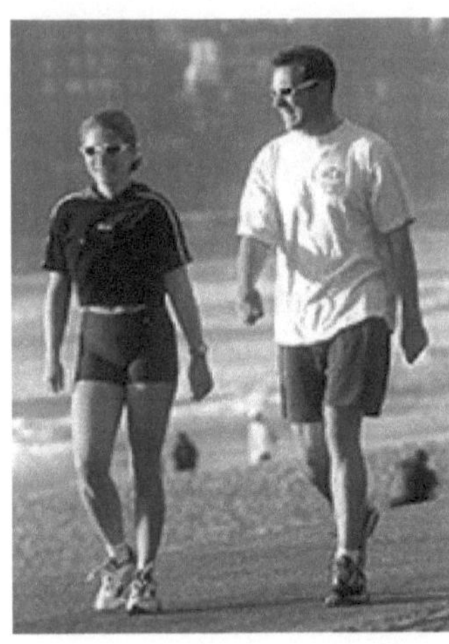

93) and lose weight. You burn about 100 calories per mile when you walk. Jogging burns about the same 100 calories per mile – but in a shorter time.   And the more you weigh, the more calories you burn during exercise.

94) Brisk walking not only helps you lose weight but also has many health benefits. So when you walk – don't saunter - walk briskly.

95) For extra exercise, park within walking distance of your destination and walk, and if you're healthy walk up stairs rather than taking an elevator or escalator.

96) For more exercise, take a brisk 15 minute walk around the mall before you start shopping.

97)   For life-long weight control take a vigorous 60 minute walk everyday! That's right – everyday. Make exercise a nonflexible top priority part of your life.

98)   To get and stay fit and help control your weight, walk everyday and work out with dumbbells for twenty minutes two or three times a week. That's all most people need.

99) Exercise key words are: consistent, persistent, dogged, unyielding, ... Get the point?

100) A common weight-loss fallacy is that you can lose abdominal fat by working your abdominal muscles. This is based on the incorrect belief that fat is eliminated from a particular part of your body if you engage the muscles underneath that layer of fat. No such luck.

101) It's a lot easier to eat 1,000 Calories than it is to burn 1,000 Calories by exercising. So a stroll after dinner won't offset the calories you ingest eating a big meal.

<u>**Bonus Tips & Secrets**</u>

102) It's much easier to stay with an exercise program when it's done in tandem, that is when you exercise with a buddy.

103)   Take a daily multi-vitamin/mineral supplement. This is important when you're on a diet – as a kind of insurance policy.

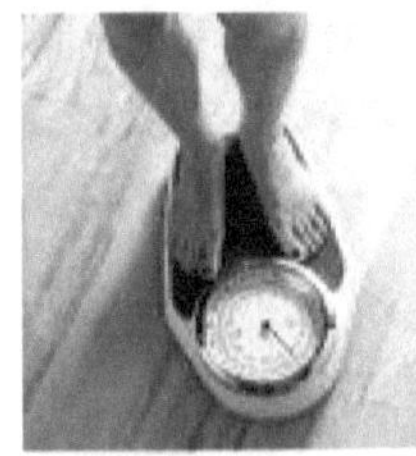

104) Weigh in once a week. There may be times when you might not see a weight loss, often because lost fat is temporarily replaced by water. This condition will gradually be corrected as you continue dieting.

105) To combat a craving think: I'm going to forgo that high-calorie dessert because I want to be around to see my children (or grandchildren) graduate from college.

106) Inevitably, you're going to be faced with a stressful situation. Instead of turning to food for comfort, be prepared with some non-food tactics that work for you, such as listening to music, reading, writing in a journal, or meditating.

107)   On a reducing diet, when you lose – you win! You win a much better chance for a longer healthier life, you win a sense of well-being, you win a more attractive appearance – and finally you win a feeling of accomplishment.

108) To prevent or delay the onset of type II diabetes, experts urge the overweight to lose weight and work out regularly. Weight loss helps your body use

insulin more efficiently, and exercise helps metabolize excess circulating blood glucose.

109) Take weight Loss one step, one meal, one workout, one day at a time.   Just think of where you'll be in a few weeks.

110) Plan to be on a diet the rest of your life. Not necessarily a weight-reducing diet.   Hopefully, at some point you'll just be maintaining your weight. But you will still need to continue to make good healthy food choices – and not slip back to your old eating habits.

111) Acquire a good low-calorie cookbook. Be sure the recipes cover breakfast, lunch and dinner, and all the recipes contain nutritional information, especially the calories per serving.

112) Obtain a comprehensive food calorie guide such as the excellent U.S.D.A. Home and Garden Bulletin No. 72: "Nutritive Value of Foods," which can be downloaded at no cost at http://www.nal.usda.gov/fnic/etext/000020.html.

113) Finally, get a scientifically sound and effective weight control book to help you lose weight in a safe and healthy manner. Consider NoPaperPress, with its extensive line of weight control, nutrition and exercise eBooks written by experts for sensible adults. No fad diets here! A list of our eBooks is on the following page.

Disclaimer

This work offers general weight control, exercise and nutrition information. It is not a medical manual and the authors do not claim to be medically qualified. The material in this book is not intended to be a substitute for medical counseling. Everyone should have a medical checkup before beginning a weight management program. Moreover, the physician conducting the medical exam should be made aware of and should approve the specific weight control program planned. Additionally, while the authors and publisher have made every effort to ensure the accuracy of the information in this book, they make no representations or warranties regarding its accuracy or completeness. Further, neither the authors nor publisher assume liability for any medical problems that might result from applying the methods in this book, or for any loss of profit, or any other commercial damages, including but not limited to special, incidental, consequential or other damages, and any such liability is hereby expressly disclaimed.

100-Day Super Diet-1200 Cal*	Weight Loss for Men - Metric*
100-Day Super Diet-1500 Cal*	Maximum Weight Loss- 1200 Cal*
100-Day No-Cooking Diet-1200 Cal*	Maximum Weight Loss- 1500 Cal*
100-Day No-Cooking Diet-1500 Cal*	Weight Control - U.S. Edition*
90-Day Smart Diet-1200 Cal*	Weight Control - Metric. Edition
90-Day Smart Diet-1500 Cal*	Professional Weight Control Women - U.S.
90-Day No-Cooking Diet - 1200 Cal*	Professional Weight Control Women - Metric
90-Day No-Cooking Diet - 1500 Cal*	Professional Weight Control Men - U.S.
90-Day Perfect Diet - 1200 Cal*	Professional Weight Control Men - Metric
90-Day Perfect Diet - 1500 Cal*	Weight Maintenance - U.S. Ed*
60-Day Perfect Diet-1200 Cal*	Weight Maintenance - Metric. Ed*
60-Day Perfect Diet-1500 Cal*	Weight Maintenance - UK Ed
50-Day Flex Diet-1200 Cal*	Weight Loss for Senior Men*
50-Day Flex Diet-1500 Cal*	Weight Loss for Senior Women*
30-Day Quick Diet - Women*	Eat Smart - U.S. Edition*
30-Day Quick Diet for Men*	Eat Smart - Metric Edition
30-Day No-Cooking Diet*	30-Day Mediterranean Diet
30-Day Diet for Women - Metric*	Exercise Smart - U.S. Edition*
30-Day Diet for Men - Metric*	Exercise Smart - Metric Edition
25 Day Easy Diet-1200 Cal*	Exercise Smart - UK Edition*
25 Day Easy Diet-1500 Cal*	Total Fitness - U.S. Edition
25-Day No-Cooking Diet	Total Fitness - Metric Edition
10-Day Express Diet	Total Fitness - UK Edition
10-Day No-Cooking Diet*	Total Fitness for Women-U.S. Ed*
7-Day Diet for Women*	Total Fitness for Women - Metric
7-Day Diet for Men*	Total Fitness for Women - UK Ed
7-Day No-Cooking Diets*	Total Fitness for Men - U.S. Ed*
90-Day Gluten-Free Diet-1200 Cal*	Total Fitness for Men- Metric Ed*
90-Day Gluten-Free Diet-1500 Cal*	Total Fitness for Men - UK Ed
30-Day Gluten-Free Quick Diet*	Senior Fitness - U.S. Edition*
30-Day Gluten-Free No-Cooking Diet*	Senior Fitness - Metric Edition*
7-Day Diet for Women - Metric*	Senior Fitness - UK Edition*
7-Day Diet for Men - Metric	Computer Diet - U.S. Edition*
7-Day Gluten-Free Express Diet*	Computer Diet - Metric Ed*
7-Day Gluten-Free No-Cooking Diet*	Reliable Weight Loss - U.S. Ed
90-Day Vegetarian Diet-1200 Cal*	101 Weight Loss Tips*
90-Day Vegetarian Diet-1500 Cal*	101 Healthy Eating Tips*
30-Day Vegetarian Diet*	101 Lifelong Fitness Tips*
7-Day Vegetarian Diet*	101 Weight Maintenance Tips
Weight Loss for Women*	101 Weight Loss Recipes
Weight Loss for Women - Metric	101 GF Weight Loss Recipes
Weight Loss for Women - UK	101 Veggie Weight Loss Recipes*
Weight Loss for Men*	30-Day Mediterranean Diet*
Maximum Weight Loss - 1200 Cal*	90-Day Mediterranean Diet - 1200 Cal*
Maximum Weight Loss - 1500 Cal*	90-Day Mediterranean Diet - 1500 Cal*

* These titles are available as both ebooks and paperbacks. Our ebooks are sold by Amazon, Apple, Google, Barnes & Noble and Kobo, but our paperbacks are only sold by Amazon

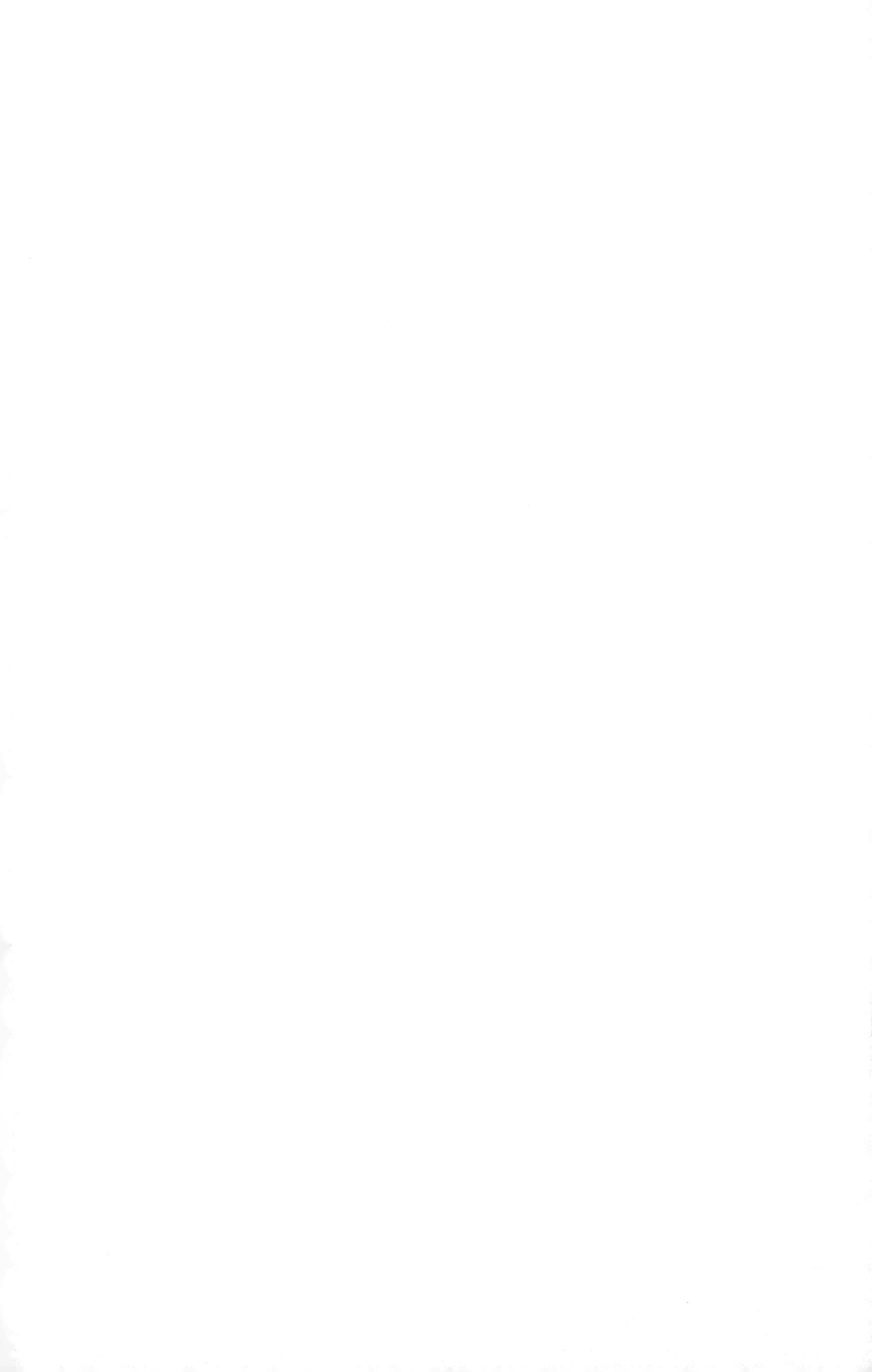

* 9 7 8 1 6 7 4 4 3 4 1 5 5 *